55 Cancer Preventing and Cancer Fighting Juice Recipes: Boost Your Immune System, Improve Your Digestion, and Become Healthier Today

By

Joseph Correa

Certified Sports Nutritionist

COPYRIGHT

ACKNOWLEDGEMENTS

The realization and success of this book could not have been possible without the motivation and support of my entire family.

55 Cancer Preventing and Cancer Fighting Juice Recipes: Boost Your Immune System, Improve Your Digestion, and Become Healthier Today

By

Joseph Correa

Certified Sports Nutritionist

CONTENTS

ABOUT THE AUTHOR

As a certified sports nutritionist, I honestly believe in the positive effects that proper nutrition can have over the body and mind. My knowledge and experience has helped me live healthier throughout the years and which I have shared with family and friends. The more you know about eating and drinking healthier, the sooner you will want to change your life and eating habits.

Nutrition is a key part in the process of being healthy and living longer so get started today.

INTRODUCTION

55 Cancer Preventing and Cancer Fighting Juice Recipes will help you to have a stronger immune system through a variety of powerful ingredients and mixtures in these juices. Cancer prevention is a serious topic that should be addressed with cardiovascular exercise, sufficient rest, and proper nutrition. These juices should not replace your normal daily meals but should complement your normal day to day meals.

Not taking the time to feed your body properly can have negative long term effects and that's why this book will save you future problems and will help teach you how to nourish your body to achieve a strong cancer fighting immune system.

This book will help you to:

-Strengthen your immune system.

-Improve your digestion.

-Cleanse Your Blood Stream.

-Have more energy.

-Become Healthier on a daily basis.

-Eliminate Toxins from your body.

Joseph Correa is a certified sports nutritionist and a professional athlete.

55 CANCER PREVENTING AND CANCER FIGHTING JUICE RECIPES

1. Beta Carotene Power

Benefits:

Beta carotene is an essential component of a healthy diet. It has been shown to reduce the risk of certain cancers, and even slows the reproduction of cancerous cells. Both cantaloupe and carrots are very high in beta-carotene. The orange adds a tasty, tangy kick to the drink and a generous dose of vitamin C.

Ingredients:

- 1/3 Cantaloupe, including rind
- 3 Carrots

- 1 Orange, peeled

How to prepare:

Wash all the ingredients thoroughly.

Juice them together and enjoy this fresh drink right away.

Total calories: 190

Vitamins: Vitamin A 15µg, Vitamin C 25mg, Calcium 10mg

Minerals: Sodium 65mg, Potassium 32 mg

Sugars 8g

2. Antioxidant Boosty

Benefits:

Nutrient dense and high in flavor, this fruity juice is sure to strengthen the immune system and help eliminate free radicals that might otherwise cause cell damage and lead to cancer. This juice recipe is a great one to try any time of the day.

Ingredients:

- 4 Apricots, pitted

- 6 large Strawberries

- 1 orange

How to prepare:

Wash all the ingredients thoroughly.

Juice them well and enjoy this fresh drink right away.

Total calories: 90

Vitamins: Vitamin A 4μg, Vitamin C 8mg, Calcium 10mg

Minerals: Sodium 32 mg, Potassium 29 mg

Sugars 4 g

3. Powerful Healer

Benefits:

Several studies have already shown that garlic, like onions or chives, reduce the risk of developing cancer of the stomach or bowel. The explanation would come from sulfur compounds contained in garlic, which would have the effect of slowing the growth of cancer cells.

Broccoli is very high in vitamin A, B, and calcium so this will lead to a healthy and strong body.

Ingredients:

- 4 large Carrots
- 4 stems of Broccoli

- 1 Garlic clove

How to prepare:

Wash all the ingredients thoroughly.

Juice them together and enjoy this fresh drink right away.

Total calories: 163

Vitamins: Vitamin A 5μg, Vitamin C 9mg, Calcium 11mg

Minerals: Sodium 15mg, Potassium 19 mg

Sugars 3 g

4. Creamery of Life

Benefits:

The high copper and vitamin C content in pears act as good anti-oxidants that can protect cells from damage by free radicals. Limonoid is a compound found in oranges that has been found to help fight cancers of the mouth, skin, lung, breast, stomach and colon.

Ingredients:

- Apples – 2, 360g

- Celery - 3 stalks, 190g

- Orange (peeled) - 125g

- Pears - 2 medium 350g

- Sweet Potato - 127g

How to prepare:

Wash all the ingredients thoroughly.

Juice them together and enjoy this fresh drink right away.

Total calories: 330

Vitamins: Vitamin A 690μg, Vitamin C 75mg, Calcium 150mg

Minerals: Sodium 152mg, Potassium 130mg

Sugars 60g

5. Carrot Mix

Benefits:

Studies have shown that lycopene, a carotenoid found in tomatoes, play a role in preventing some types of cancers like lung, prostate and colon cancer. Carrots do wonders for boosting the immune system, they increase the performance of white blood cells and also help eliminate excess fluids from the body. Carrots reduce the risk of stroke by 68% and the risk of lung cancer by 50%. It increases immunity through beta-carotene which it contains in large quantities.

Ingredients:

- Carrots - 144g

- Celery - 3 stalks, 192g

- Cucumber - 1/2 cucumber 150g

- Parsley - 2 handful 80g

- Tomatoes - 3 medium whole 365g

How to prepare:

Wash all the ingredients thoroughly.

Juice them together and enjoy this fresh drink right away.

Total calories: 90

Vitamins: Vitamin A 980µg, Vitamin C 150mg, Calcium 211mg

Minerals: Sodium 235mg, Potassium 190mg

Sugars 16g

6. Sweet Grapefruit

Benefits:

Ginger has been tested and it has been shown that it might slow and even prevent cancerous tumor growth. The anti-oxidant in oranges helps the skin from free radical damage and also reduces the risk of heart disease.

Ingredients:

- Cranberries - 3 cups, 290g

- Ginger Root - 45g

- Grapefruit (peeled) 400g

- Oranges - 3 fruits 350g

How to prepare:

Wash all the ingredients thoroughly.

Juice them together and enjoy this fresh drink right away.

Total calories: 213

Vitamins: Vitamin A 124μg, Vitamin C 210mg, Calcium 140mg

Minerals: Sodium 10mg, Potassium 130mg

Sugars 51g

7. Super Strawberry Time

Benefits:

Strawberry helps lower cancer death rates, because of the high content of various anti-oxidants that prevent damage caused by free radicals in our body, and they also detoxify the body. It has been shown that apple skin extract lowers the risks of colon and liver cancer.

Ingredients:

- Apples - 2 large 440g

- Lemon - 1/2 fruit 32g

- Strawberries - 3 cups, 430g

How to prepare:

Wash all the ingredients thoroughly.

Juice them together and enjoy this fresh drink right away.

Total calories: 190

Vitamins: Vitamin A 9µg, Vitamin C 180mg, Calcium 71mg

Minerals: Sodium 5mg, Potassium 790mg

Sugars 45g

8. Green Mile Mix

Benefits:

Consuming vitamin C helps lower the incidence of peptic ulcers and reduces the risk of stomach cancer. The carotene found in spinach is beneficial in fighting and preventing cancer and is a powerful anti-oxidant and anti-cancer agent. The high content of iron in spinach makes it a great blood builder and it supplies fresh oxygen for the whole body.

Ingredients:

- Brussel Sprout – 1 sprout 17g

- Cucumber -1, 300g

- Oranges - 2, 260g

- Pineapple – ¼ 225g

- Spinach – 4 handful 102g

How to prepare:

Wash all the ingredients thoroughly.

Juice them together and enjoy this fresh drink right away.

Total calories: 180

Vitamins: Vitamin A 430µg, Vitamin C 209mg, Calcium 215mg

Minerals: Sodium 74mg, Potassium 130mg, Sugars 34g

9. Coconut PO Mix

Benefits:

Oranges being high in vitamin C reduce the risk of heart diseases, and reduce the risk of stomach cancer. Coconuts might play an important role in reducing all types of cancer risk.

Ingredients:

- Coconut (meat only) - 1 medium 390g

- Oranges - 2 large 365g

- Peaches - 2 medium 300g

How to prepare:

Wash all the ingredients thoroughly.

Juice them together and enjoy this fresh drink right away.

Total calories: 950

Vitamins: Vitamin A 59μg, Vitamin C 156mg, Calcium 148mg

Minerals: Sodium 53mg, Potassium 180mg

Sugars 53g

10. Pineapple Peppermint Combo

Benefits:

The high content of vitamin C in pears make it a good source of anti-oxidants that can protect cell damage by free radicals. They are also high in fructose and glucose, so you get a natural boost of energy. Strawberries can help improve memory, concentration, and the brain's ability to process information.

Ingredients:

- Pear - 1 medium 175g

- Peppermint - 0.75g

- Pineapple - ½ 450g

- Strawberry - 1 cup, 140g

How to prepare:

Wash all the ingredients thoroughly.

Juice them together and enjoy this fresh drink right away.

Total calories: 220

Vitamins: Vitamin A 11μg, Vitamin C 214mg, Calcium 67mg

Minerals: Sodium 4mg, Potassium 612mg

Sugars 41g

11. ACG Juice

Benefits:

Limonoid is a compound found in oranges that fights cancer of the mouth, skin, lung, stomach and breast. Ginger has been proven to help prevent cancerous tumor growth, and let's not forget apples play an role to in preventing cancer too.

Ingredients:

- Apples - 3 medium 540g

- Celery - 4 stalks, large 255g

- Ginger Root - 1/4 thumb 6g

- Lemon (with rind) - 1/2 fruit 30g

- Orange (peeled) - 1 large 181g

How to prepare:

Wash all the ingredients thoroughly.

Juice them together and enjoy this fresh drink right away.

Total calories: 211

Vitamins: Vitamin A 420µg, Vitamin C 120mg, Calcium 200mg

Minerals: Sodium 201mg, Potassium 1520 mg,

Sugars 54g

12. Green Friend

Benefits:

Bell peppers are powerful anti-oxidants, helpful in preventing cancers of the pancreas and prostate. Tomatoes are a good source of melatonin that protects again breast cancer in many ways.

Ingredients:

- Apples (green) - 2 medium 360g

- Carrots - 3 medium 180g

- Cucumber - 1 cucumber 300g

- Grapes (green) - 15 grapes 90g

- Pepper (sweet green) - 1 medium 115g

- Tomato - 1 medium whole (2-3/5" dia) 120g

How to prepare:

Wash all the ingredients thoroughly.

Juice them together and enjoy this fresh drink right away.

Total calories: 220

Vitamins: Vitamin A 1290μg, Vitamin C 150mg, Calcium 150mg

Minerals: Sodium 132mg, Potassium 1654mg

Sugars: 39

13. T Life

Benefits:

Large quantities of potassium helps relieve the symptoms of stress. Several antioxidant substances are contained in tomato juice, including lycopene that help prevent damage caused by free radicals to body tissues.

Ingredients:

- Basil (dried) - 1 dash, ground 0.17g

- Cauliflower - 1/2 head medium 294g

- Cucumber - 1 cucumber 301g

- Tomatoes - 2 cups cherry tomatoes 298g

- Apple- 1, 180g

How to prepare:

Wash all the ingredients thoroughly.

Juice them together and enjoy this fresh drink right away.

Total calories: 100

Vitamins: Vitamin A 101µg, Vitamin C 130mg, Calcium 98mg

Minerals: Sodium 74g, Potassium 140g

Sugars 11g

14. Broccoli Power

Benefits:

Vitamin C and certain amino acids make broccoli a very good detoxifier. Free radicals are eliminated from the body and the blood is purified. Broccoli reduces risk of breast and uterus cancers as it removes extra estrogen form the body. It also contains antioxidants and fibers.

Ingredients:

- Apple - 1 medium 182g

- Blueberries - 1 cup 148g

- Broccoli - 1 stalk 151g

- Carrots - 3 large 210g

How to prepare:

Wash all the ingredients thoroughly.

Juice them together and enjoy this fresh drink right away.

Total calories: 202

Vitamins: Vitamin A 230µg, Vitamin C 110mg, Calcium 150mg

Minerals: Sodium 220mg, Potassium 140mg

Sugars 40g

15. The 3 Way

Benefits:

Eating an apple a day can reduce the risk of breast cancer and lower the risk of colon cancer. Being high in vitamin C, oranges help stimulate white cells to fight infections.

Ingredients:

- Apples - 4 medium 720g

- Celery - 2 stalks, large 125g

- Oranges (peeled) - 2 fruit 261g

How to prepare:

Wash all the ingredients thoroughly.

Juice them together and enjoy this fresh drink right away.

Total calories: 320

Vitamins: Vitamin A 51µg, Vitamin C 125mg, Calcium 140mg

Minerals: Sodium 71mg, Potassium 112mg

Sugars 76g

16. Beet Mix

Benefits:

Carrots reduce cholesterol levels and the chance of having a heart attack. Beetroot is a treatment used for leukemia in some countries. They contain an amino acid called betaine that has anti-cancer properties.

Ingredients:

- Apple - 1 medium 180g

- Beetroot - 1 beet) 175g

- Carrots - 10 medium 630g

- Lemon - 1/2 fruit 42g

- Kiwi (peeled) - 2 fruits 260g

How to prepare:

Wash all the ingredients thoroughly.

Juice them together and enjoy this fresh drink right away.

Total calories: 320

Vitamins: Vitamin A 3900µg, Vitamin C 160mg, Calcium 250mg

Minerals: Sodium 430mg, Potassium 230mg

Sugars 60g

17. Apple-Spinach Combo

Benefits:

Spinach can slow down cancerous cell division, especially in cancers of the breast, cervical, prostate, stomach, and skin. Pears have a high amount of fructose, which helps you get a quick and natural boost of energy.

Ingredients:

- Apple - 1 medium 180g

- Carrots - 5 medium 304g

- Cucumber - 1 cucumber 300g

- Pear - 1 medium 175g

- Spinach - 2 handful 50g

How to prepare:

- **Wash all the ingredients thoroughly.**

- **Juice them together and enjoy this fresh drink right away.**

Total calories: 210

Vitamins: Vitamin A 1850µg, Vitamin C 58mg, Calcium 165mg

Minerals: Sodium 150mg, Potassium 130mg

Sugars 39g

18. Exotic Sulforaphane Juice

Benefits:

Sulforaphane from Kale has been shown to have a more direct effect on cancer prevention, especially in colon cancer, inducing cancer cells to destroy themselves. Ginger helps reduce inflammation, so it can be used to treat any disease.

Ingredients:

- Ginger Root - 1/2 thumb 12g

- Kale - 4 leaves 140g

- Mango - 1 fruit 335g

- Pineapple - 1 cup, chunks 165g

How to prepare:

Wash all the ingredients thoroughly.

Juice them together and enjoy this fresh drink right away.

Total calories: 219

Vitamins: Vitamin A 619µg, Vitamin C 250mg, Calcium 216mg

Minerals: Sodium 35mg, Potassium 101mg

Sugars 48g

19. Red Mango Breakfast

Benefits:

Beta-carotene consumption has been linked to reduced risks of several cancers, notably lung cancer. Strawberries can actually be helpful to thin blood and prevent blood clots formation, thereby reducing the work of the heart

Ingredients:

- Apples - 2 medium 362g

- Cabbage (red) - 2 leaves 46g

- Carrots - 3 medium 180g

- Mango (peeled) - 1 fruit 336g

- Strawberries - 1.5 cup, whole 216g

How to prepare:

Wash all the ingredients thoroughly.

Juice them together and enjoy this fresh drink right away.

Total calories: 230

Vitamins: Vitamin A 1300µg, Vitamin C 141mg, Calcium 192mg

Minerals: Sodium 242mg, Potassium 1328mg

Sugars 20g

20. Kiwi Kick

Benefits:

Strawberries can improve memory and the brain's ability to process information, and they also detoxify the body. Nutrients contained in kiwifruit have antioxidant properties as well.

Ingredients:

- Blueberries - 2 cups 290g

- Kiwifruit - 2 fruits 135g

- Peppermint - 50 leaves 2.5g

- Strawberries - 16 medium 190g

How to prepare:

Wash all the ingredients thoroughly.

Juice them together and enjoy this fresh drink right away.

Total calories: 175

Vitamins: Vitamin A 13µg, Vitamin C 170mg, Calcium 65mg

Minerals: Sodium 5mg, Potassium 620mg

Sugars 3g

21. Blackberry Rain

Benefits:

Pears have anti-oxidants and anti-carcinogen which help prevent high blood pressure. Consuming vitamin C rich foods helps to lower the incidence of peptic ulcers and in turn, reduces the risk of stomach cancer.

Ingredients:

- Blackberry - 1 cup 140g

- Kiwifruit - 1 fruit 65g

- Pear - 1 medium 175g

- Pineapple (peeled, cored) - 1/4 fruit 220g

How to prepare:

Wash all the ingredients thoroughly.

Juice them together and enjoy this fresh drink right away.

Total calories: 150

Vitamins: Vitamin A 19μg, Vitamin C 135mg, Calcium 71mg

Minerals: Sodium 5mg, Potassium 610mg

Sugars 35g

22. Kale Fighter

Benefits:

Collards are rich in invaluable sources of phyto-nutrients with potent anti-cancer properties, such as diindolylmethane (DIM) and sulforaphane that have proven benefits against prostate, breast cancer.

Ingredients:

- Apple - 1 medium 182g

- Collard Greens - 1 cup, chopped 36g

- Kale - 4 leaves (8-12") 140g

- Pepper (sweet red) - 1 medium 119g

How to prepare:

Wash all the ingredients thoroughly.

Juice them together and enjoy this fresh drink right away.

Total calories: 110

Vitamins: Vitamin A 1400μg, Vitamin C 192mg, Calcium 180mg

Minerals: Sodium 103mg, Potassium 124mg

Sugars 18g

23. Golden Lemon Energy

Benefits:

According to a study of 20,000 people, those who ate the most apples had 40 percent lower risk of developing lung cancer. The high content of vitamin K is essential in anchoring calcium in bones, making it important to bone health.

Ingredients:

- Apples - 2 medium 360g

- Cucumber - 1/2 cucumber 150g

- Lemon - 1 fruit 65g

- Spinach - 5 cups 150g

How to prepare:

Wash all the ingredients thoroughly.

Juice them together and enjoy this fresh drink right away.

Total calories: 140

Vitamins: Vitamin A 490µg, Vitamin C 51mg, Calcium 140mg

Minerals: Sodium 85mg, Potassium 980mg

Sugars 25g

24. Healthy Triple P

Benefits:

Research found an extract from apple skin extract which had a 57 percent lowering effect on liver cancer risk. Extracts from parsley have been used in animal studies to help increase the antioxidant capacity of the blood.

Ingredients:

- Apple - 1/2 medium 90g

- Cucumber - 1/2 cucumber 150.5g

- Ginger Root - 1 thumb24g

- Papaya (deseeded) - 1/4 fruit, 195.25g

- Parsley - 1 handful 40g

- Pear - 1/2 medium 89g

How to prepare:

Wash all the ingredients thoroughly.

Juice them together and enjoy this fresh drink right away.

Total calories: 125

Vitamins: Vitamin A 251µg, Vitamin C 120mg, Calcium 122mg

Minerals: Sodium 65mg, Potassium 700mg

Sugars 20g

25. Let Us Help You

Benefits:

Lettuce juice is an excellent source of hydration at the cellular level. It is also rich in anti-oxidants especially beta-carotene, vitamin C and vitamin E. These substances help prevent premature aging.

Ingredients:

- Apples - 2 medium 360g

- Celery - 2 stalks, large 125g

- Cucumber - 1/2 cucumber 150g

- Lettuce - 2 cups 94g

How to prepare:

Wash all the ingredients thoroughly.

Juice them together and enjoy this fresh drink right away.

Total calories: 154

Vitamins: Vitamin A 320µg, Vitamin C 61mg, Calcium 125mg

Minerals: Sodium 76mg, Potassium 874mg

Sugars 34g

26. Sweet Blend

Benefits:

The pigment that gives beets their rich, purple-crimson color is also a powerful cancer-fighting agent. Research shows that beet juice can help inhibit the development of colon and stomach cancer.

Ingredients:

- Apples (golden delicious) – 2, 364g

- Beetroots - 2 beets 164g

- Carrot - 1 large 72g

- Sweet Potato - 1 , 130g

How to prepare:

Wash all the ingredients thoroughly.

Juice them together and enjoy this fresh drink right away.

Total calories: 234

Vitamins: Vitamin A 986μg, Vitamin C 155mg, Calcium 110mg

Minerals: Sodium 156mg, Potassium 1390mg

Sugars 41g

27. Melon World

Benefits:

Lycopene (from red watermelons) has been extensively researched for its anti-oxidant and cancer-preventing properties. It is especially helpful to fight prostate cancer.

Ingredients:

Tomato - 1 medium whole 120g

Watermelon - 1 large wedge 570g

How to prepare:

Wash all the ingredients thoroughly.

Juice them together and enjoy this fresh drink right away.

Total calories: 109

Vitamins: Vitamin A 142µg, Vitamin C 41mg, Calcium 31mg

Minerals: Sodium 6mg, Potassium 620mg

Sugars 22g

28. Fruit Dance

Benefits:

The abundant content of vitamin A and carotenoids help prevent age-related eye problems. A research shows that the pectin in apples reduces the risk of colon cancer and helps maintain a healthy digestive tract. This juice is also an antioxidant, it strengthens the immune system, aids digestion, and it is diuretic.

Ingredients:

- Apples - 2 medium 360g

- Avocado - 1 avocado 200g

- Celery - 3 stalks, large 190g

- Grapes - 15 grapes 90g

- Spinach - 2 cups 60g

How to prepare:

Wash all the ingredients thoroughly.

Juice them together and enjoy this fresh drink right away.

Total calories: 320

Vitamins: Vitamin A 235µg, Vitamin C 51mg, Calcium 143mg

Minerals: Sodium 139mg, Potassium 1690mg

Sugars 28g

29. Carrot Path

Benefits:

Studies show that women who ate raw carrots were five to eight times less likely to develop breast cancer than women who did not eat carrots. Pectin in carrots lowers the serum cholesterol levels.

Ingredients:

- Apple - 1 medium 182g

- Carrots - 3 medium 182g

- Garlic - 2 cloves 6g

- Ginger Root - 1 thumb 24g

How to prepare:

Wash all the ingredients thoroughly.

Juice them together and enjoy this fresh drink right away.

Total calories: 98

Vitamins: Vitamin A 1083µg, Vitamin C 47mg, Calcium 82mg

Minerals: Sodium 97mg, Potassium 705mg

Sugars 15g

30. KL Juice

Benefits:

Kale is a rich source of organ sulfur compounds, which is great at fighting many cancers. Recent studies show that ginger might also have a role in lowering LDL cholesterol because the spice can help reduce the amount of cholesterol that is absorbed.

Ingredients:

- Celery - 4 stalks, large 256g
- Cucumber - 1 cucumber 301g
- Ginger Root - 1 thumb 24g
- Kale - 6 leaves 210g

How to prepare:

- **Wash all the ingredients thoroughly.**

- **Juice them together and enjoy this fresh drink right away.**

Total calories: 220

Vitamins: Vitamin A 200μg, Vitamin C 99mg, Calcium 34mg

Minerals: Sodium 12mg, Potassium 64mg

Sugars 10g

31. Lemon Topping

Benefits:

Beetroot is a treatment used for leukemia because it contains an amino acid called betaine. Drinking lemon juice is helpful for people suffering from heart problems, as it contains potassium which controls blood pressure.

Ingredients:

- Beetroot - 1 beet 175g

- Cabbage (red) - 2 leaves 46g

- Carrots - 3 medium 183g

- Lime - 1/2 fruit 42g

- Orange - 1 fruit 131g

- Apple – 1 180g

How to prepare:

Wash all the ingredients thoroughly.

Juice them together and enjoy this fresh drink right away.

Total calories: 296

Vitamins: Vitamin A 500μg, Vitamin C 152mg, Calcium 52mg

Minerals: Sodium 40mg, Potassium 190mg

Sugars 19g

32. Fiesta Cocktail

Benefits:

Oranges being high in flavonoids reduce the risk of heart disease and also build a strong immune system. Their vitamin C content acts as a good anti-oxidant which protects cells from free radical damage.

Ingredients:

- Apples - 2 medium 360g

- Celery - 2 stalks, medium) 80g

- Cucumber - 1 cucumber 301g

- Lemon - 1/2 fruit 42g

- Oranges (peeled) - 2 fruits 260g

How to prepare:

Wash all the ingredients thoroughly.

Juice them together and enjoy this fresh drink right away.

Total calories: 190

Vitamins: Vitamin A 48μg, Vitamin C 98mg, Calcium 40mg

Minerals: Sodium 19mg, Potassium 101mg

Sugars: 12g

33. Orange Banana Life

Benefits:

Apples are great, because they really reduce the risk of any type of cancer, and oranges have a high content of vitamin C that helps your immune system get stronger.

Ingredients:

- Apple - 1 medium 180g

- Cucumber - 1 cucumber (301g

- Orange - 1 large 154g

- Banana- 1 medium 150 g

How to prepare:

Wash all the ingredients thoroughly.

Juice them together and enjoy this fresh drink right away.

Total calories: 215

Vitamins: Vitamin A 20μg, Vitamin C 70mg, Calcium 79mg,

Minerals: Sodium 156, Potassium 900mg

Sugars 25g

34. BOA Time

Benefits:

Apples protect the body from free radicals effects, and oranges are well known for reducing cancer risk. Bananas are high in potassium as well.

Ingredients:

- Apple – 1 large 213g

- Orange (peeled) - 1 fruit without refuse 316g

- Banana (peeled) – 1 medium 150 g

How to prepare:

Wash all the ingredients thoroughly.

Juice them together and enjoy this fresh drink right away.

Total calories: 209

Vitamins: Vitamin A 110µg, Vitamin C 64mg, Calcium 30mg

Minerals: Sodium 49mg, Potassium 390mg

Sugars 7g

35. Lemony Mango Kicker

Benefits:

Lemons are a great way of maintaining your body healthy and help prevent skin cancer. Mangos reduce colon and breast cancer.

Ingredients:

- Apples - 1 medium 180g

- Lemon (peeled) - 1/2 fruit 25g

- Mango (peeled) – 1/2 fruit 70 g

How to prepare:

Wash all the ingredients thoroughly.

Juice them together and enjoy this fresh drink right away.

Total calories: 90

Vitamins: Vitamin A 420µg, Vitamin C 14.9mg, Calcium 20mg,

Minerals: Sodium 12mg, Potassium 230mg

Sugars 4g

36. Apple Lime Combo

Benefits:

Cabbage keeps blood pressure from getting high and allows you to control it better. Pears are high in nutrients and prevent many types of cancer.

Ingredients:

- Apple- 1 medium 180 g

- Cabbage (red) - 2 leaves 52g

- Lime - 1/2 fruit 27g

- Pears - 2 medium 346g

How to prepare:

Wash all the ingredients thoroughly.

Juice them together and enjoy this fresh drink right away.

Total calories: 205

Vitamins: Vitamin A 29µg, Vitamin C 48.1mg, Calcium 40mg

Minerals: Sodium 12mg, Potassium 400mg

Sugars 5g

37. Pearing World

Benefits:

Pears are a great way of building up your immune system, and lemons, due to their high content of Vitamin C, are very rich in antioxidants which prevent cancer by keeping the immune system strong.

Ingredients:

- Lemon (peeled) – ½ fruit 25g

- Pears- 1 medium 170g

- Spinach – 2 handful 50g

- Banana – 2 medium 300g

How to prepare:

Wash all the ingredients thoroughly.

Juice them together and enjoy this fresh drink right away.

Total calories: 190

Vitamins: Vitamin A 210µg, Vitamin C 83mg, Calcium 150mg,

Minerals: Sodium 33mg, Potassium 230mg

Sugars 8g

38. Morning Beet Surprise

Benefits:

Apples are powerful natural antioxidants. It has been shown that apple skin extract lowers the risks of colon and liver cancer. Beetroot fights inflammation and can also improve vision.

Ingredients:

- Apple - 1 medium 180g

- Beetroot - 1/2 beet 40g

- Orange (peeled) - 1 medium 140 g

- Spinach- 1 handful 25g

How to prepare:

Wash all the ingredients thoroughly.

Juice them together and enjoy this fresh drink right away.

Total calories: 84

Vitamins: Vitamin A 300µg, Vitamin C 19mg, Calcium 21mg,

Minerals: Sodium 30mg, Potassium 218mg

Sugars 5g

39. Grape Celery Combo

Benefits:

Bananas are great for supporting heart health, oranges can reduce cancer risks and celery contains good salts. Limonoid is a compound found in oranges that has been found to help fight cancers of the mouth, skin, lung, breast, stomach and colon.

Ingredients:

- Banana (peeled) – 1 medium 150g

- Celery – 2stalks, 142g

- Grapes – 14 grapes 80g

- Orange- 1 medium 140

How to prepare:

Wash all the ingredients thoroughly.

Juice them together and enjoy this fresh drink right away.

Total calories: 90

Vitamins: Vitamin A 108μg, Vitamin C 40mg, Calcium 80mg

Minerals: Sodium 30mg, Potassium 100mg

Sugars 4g

40. PAC Punch

Benefits:

Apples reduce risk of cancer, peaches are high in nutrients and vitamins, and carrots are a great source of beta-carotene. Carrots increase the performance of white blood cells and also help eliminate excess fluids from the body.

Ingredients:

- Peaches - 3medium   450g
- Apple -1 medium 180 g
- Carrots- 2/80g

How to prepare:

Wash all the ingredients thoroughly.

Juice them together and enjoy this fresh drink right away.

Total calories: 352

Vitamins: Vitamin A 600uq, Vitamin C 45mg, Calcium 40mg,

Minerals: Sodium 12mg, Potassium 310mg

Sugars 6g

41. Double Beet

Benefits:

Parsley and Tomatoes are high in antioxidants and also play a role in regulating high blood pressure and let's not forget that carrots reduce the risk of cancer.

Ingredients:

- Beetroot - 1 beet 81g

- Carrots – 1 medium 60g

- Celery - 2 stalks, large 125g

- Parsley - 4 handful 160g

- Tomatoes-2 120g

How to prepare:

Wash all the ingredients thoroughly.

Juice them together and enjoy this fresh drink right away.

Total calories: 203

Vitamins: Vitamin A 1273µg, Vitamin C 200.4mg, Calcium

Minerals: Sodium 44mg, Potassium 62mg

Sugars 21 g

42. C Plus

Benefits:

Ginger helps slow or even prevent cancerous tumor growth and the pectin in carrots lowers the serum cholesterol levels

Ingredients:

- Carrots - 3 large 215g

- Celery - 4 stalks, large 255g

- Cucumber - 1/2 cucumber 150g

- Ginger Root - 1/2 thumb 11g

- Apple-1 medium 80 g

How to prepare:

Wash all the ingredients thoroughly.

Juice them together and enjoy this fresh drink right away.

Total calories: 141

Vitamins: Vitamin A 1201µg, Vitamin C 17mg, Calcium 150mg

Minerals: Sodium 270mg, Potassium 1307mg

Sugars 23g

43. CAB Mix

Benefits:

Apples reduce cholesterol and the risk of many types of cancer. Some studies regarding cucumber have shown that they might control the speed that cancer cells multiply at.

Ingredients:

- Apples - 1 medium 180g

- Beetroot - 1 beet 80g

- Cucumber- 135g

How to prepare:

Wash all the ingredients thoroughly.

Juice them together and enjoy this fresh drink right away.

Total calories: 165

Vitamins: Vitamin A 603μg, Vitamin C 17mg, Calcium 40mg

Minerals: Sodium 95mg, Potassium 750

Sugars 30g

44. Cancer Fighter

Benefits:

Apples are great to detoxify your liver. The extract from apple skins can lower risk of liver cancer and other cancers.

Ingredients:

- Apple - 1 medium 180g

- Grapes - 80g

- Carrots - 2 large 140g

- Lime- 1 fruit 60 g

How to prepare:

Wash all the ingredients thoroughly.

Juice them together and enjoy this fresh drink right away.

Total calories: 95

Vitamins: Vitamin A 707μg. Vitamin C 17mg, Calcium 55mg

Minerals: Copper: Sodium 125mg, Potassium 603mg

Sugars 22g

45. Jungle Green

Benefits:

1 apple per day reduces risk of cancer. Lemons are great for fighting all types of cancers and immune system deficiencies.

Ingredients:

- Bitter Melon - 1 bitter melon 110g

- Mango - 1/2 large 160g

- Lemon (with peel) - 1 fruit 80g

- Apple- 1 medium 80g

How to prepare:

Wash all the ingredients thoroughly.

Juice them together and enjoy this fresh drink right away.

Total calories: 55

Vitamins: Vitamin A 78μg, Vitamin C 157mg, Calcium 49mg

Minerals: Sodium 43mg, Potassium 81mg

Sugars 12g

46. Triple C

Benefits:

Celery is well known for his high antioxidant content, and cilantro is very good for maintaining strong bones and a powerful immune system which essential when fighting cancer.

Ingredients:

- Carrot – 3 medium 180g

- Celery - 2 stalks, large 120g

- Cilantro - 1 handful 32g

- Apple -1 medium 80g

How to prepare:

Wash all the ingredients thoroughly.

Juice them together and enjoy this fresh drink right away.

Total calories: 20

Vitamins: Vitamin A 336µg, Vitamin C 18.2mg, Calcium 80

Minerals: Sodium 25mg, Potassium 120mg

Sugars 5g

47. Light Mix

Benefits:

Beets are high in carbohydrates which means they are a great instant energy source. Research also shows that beet juice can help inhibit the development of colon cancer and lime is a natural antiseptic.

Ingredients:

- Apple - 1 medium 180g

- Beetroot - 1 beet 80g

- Lime - 1/2 fruit 29g

- Spinach- 2 cup 60g

How to prepare:

Wash all the ingredients thoroughly.

Juice them together and enjoy this fresh drink right away.

Total calories: 179

Vitamins: Vitamin A 9µg, Vitamin C 101mg, Calcium 50mg

Minerals: Sodium 45mg, Potassium 625mg

Sugars 36g

48. Banana on Top

Benefits:

Tomato juice has anti-oxidant and diuretic properties and also improves digestive functions. It also helps detoxify the liver and kidneys. Apples reduce the risk of liver cancer.

Ingredients:

- Apples - 2 medium 350g

- Cucumber - 1 cucumber 300g

- Spinach - 2 cups 60g

- Tomato - 1 medium whole 115g

- Banana-1 medium 150g

How to prepare:

Wash all the ingredients thoroughly.

Juice them together and enjoy this fresh drink right away.

Total calories: 190

Vitamins: Vitamin A 1012μg, Vitamin C 98mg, Calcium 150mg

Minerals: Sodium 129mg, Potassium 1505mg

Sugars 31g

49. Tomato Flow

Benefits:

Tomatoes contain another powerful anti-inflammatory agents, which are particularly concentrated in the tomato skin. This fights inflammation and it may play a role in the prevention of some types of cancer.

Ingredients:

- Celery - 1 stalk, large 60g

- Cilantro - 1 handful 35g

- Garlic - 1 clove 3g

- Tomato - 1 cup cherry tomatoes 145g

How to prepare:

Wash all the ingredients thoroughly.

Juice them together and enjoy this fresh drink right away.

Total calories: 30

Vitamins: Vitamin A 151µg, Vitamin C 86mg,

Minerals: Sodium 140mg, Potassium 620mg

Sugars 5g

50. Limonoid Check

Benefits:

It is well known that limonoids in lemons inhibit the development of cancer, and apples reduce the risk of having cancer.

Ingredients:

- Apples – 3 medium 545g

- Celery - 3 stalks, large 190g

- Grapes- 70g

- Lemon (peeled) - 1 fruit 58g

How to prepare:

Wash all the ingredients thoroughly.

Juice them together and enjoy this fresh drink right away.

Total calories: 212

Vitamins: Vitamin A 679μg, Vitamin C 131.4mg, Calcium 230mg

Minerals: Sodium 179mg, Potassium 1430mg

Sugars 51g

51. Mango Ginger

Benefits:

A flavonoid called hesperidin found in oranges can lower high blood pressure and prevent cancer. Ginger has been proven to help prevent cancerous tumor growth.

Ingredients:

- Ginger Root - 1/2 thumb 10g

- Grapes: 140g

- Mango - 1 fruit without refuse 330g

- Orange - 1 small 95g

- Pineapple - 1 cup, chunks 165g

How to prepare:

Wash all the ingredients thoroughly.

Juice them together and enjoy this fresh drink right away.

Total calories: 230

Vitamins: Vitamin A 625µg, Vitamin C 294.2mg, Calcium 201mg

Minerals: Sodium 40mg, Potassium 1104mg

Sugars: 4g

52. Ginger Pineapple Delight

Benefits:

Pineapple reduces risk of progression of age-related macular degeneration. Ginger Root is great as it prevents cancerous tumor growth and can also help knock out a high fever.

Ingredients:

- Ginger Root - 1/2 thumb 10g

- Mango - 1 fruit without refuse 335g

- Orange - 1 small 95g

- Pineapple - 1 cup, chunks 165g

How to prepare:

Wash all the ingredients thoroughly.

Juice them together and enjoy this fresh drink right away.

Total calories: 212

Vitamins: Vitamin A 536µg, Vitamin C 328.1mg, Calcium 321mg,

Minerals: Sodium 39mg, Potassium 1088mg

Sugars 44g

53. Sweet Greens

Benefits:

Apples protect brain cells from free radical damage, and broccoli reduces all types of cancers. Sulforaphane from Kale has been shown to have a powerful effect on cancer prevention, especially in colon cancer, inducing cancer cells to destroy themselves.

Ingredients:

- Apple - 1 medium 180g

- Broccoli - 150g

- Collard Greens - 1 cup, chopped 35g

- Kale - 4 leaves (8-12") 140g

- Orange-1, 135 g

How to prepare:

Wash all the ingredients thoroughly.

Juice them together and enjoy this fresh drink right away.

Total calories: 158

Vitamins: Vitamin A 650μg, Vitamin C 213mg, Calcium 180

Minerals: Sodium 126mg, Potassium 953mg

Sugars 21g

54. Dande Mix

Benefits:

Dandelion Greens are very well known for the fact that they reduce the risk of cancer and lowers stress levels. Lemons are a great source of vitamin C that helps the body maintain a strong immune system.

Ingredients:

- Apples - 2 medium 360g

- Cucumber - 1/2 cucumber 150g

- Dandelion Greens - 1 cup, chopped 55g

- Lemon - 1/2 fruit 42g

- Sweet potato- 120g

How to prepare:

Wash all the ingredients thoroughly.

Juice them together and enjoy this fresh drink right away.

Total calories: 178

Vitamins: Vitamin A 531µg, Vitamin C 130mg, Calcium 200mg,

Minerals: Sodium 95mg, Potassium 1013mg

Sugars 25g

55. ABP Start

Benefits:

Apples are very good because they reduce the risk of cancer. Bell peppers are powerful anti-oxidants, helpful in preventing cancers of the pancreas and prostate.

Ingredients:

- Apples - 2 medium 350g

- Beetroots - 2 beets 160

- Carrot- 1/ 65g

- Pepper (sweet red) - 1 medium 115g

How to prepare:

Wash all the ingredients thoroughly.

Juice them together and enjoy this fresh drink right away.

Total calories: 230

Vitamins: Vitamin A 970µg, Vitamin C 124mg, Calcium 103mg,

Minerals: Sodium 10 mg, Potassium 231 mg

Sugars 6g

Other Great Titles by This Author

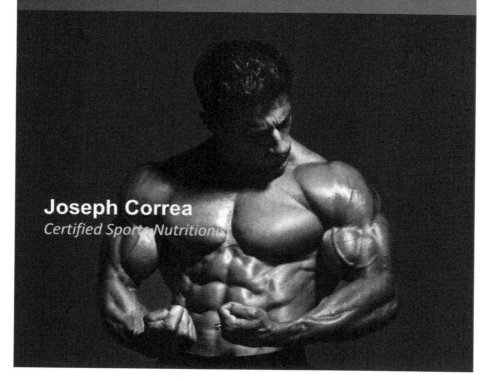

45

Muscle Building Recipes
to Gain Muscle Mass
Without Shakes or Pills
High Protein Content in
Every Meal!

Joseph Correa
Certified Sports Nutritionist

35
Diabetic Meal
Recipes

The Most Delicious Way to Stay Healthy

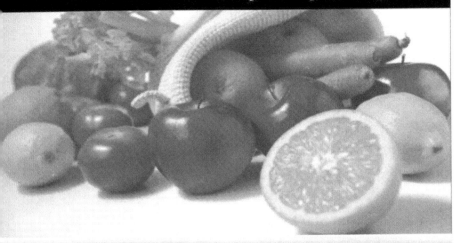

Joseph Correa
Certified Sports Nutritionist

95 MEAL AND JUICE RECIPES FOR **DIABETICS:**

A DAILY NUTRITION RECIPE BOOK FOR PEOPLE WITH DIABETES

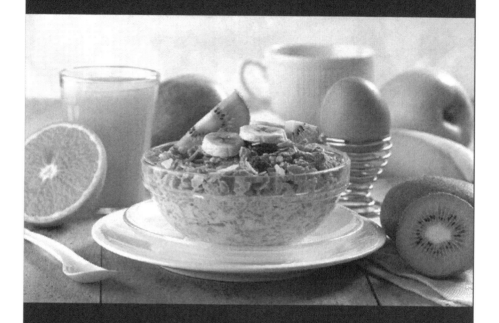

Joseph Correa

Certified Sports Nutritionist

170

MEAL AND JUICE RECIPES
TO **LOSE WEIGHT**
AND LOWER YOUR HIGH BLOOD PRESSURE:

THE **PERFECT SOLUTION**
TO YOUR **HEALTH PROBLEMS**

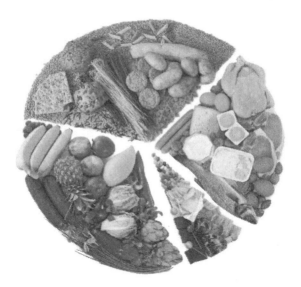

Joseph Correa

Certified Sports Nutritionist

50 WEIGHT LOSS JUICES RECIPES FOR BODY CLEANSING:

LOSE WEIGHT FAST BEFORE YOUR WEDDING, PARTY, OR SPECIAL EVENT

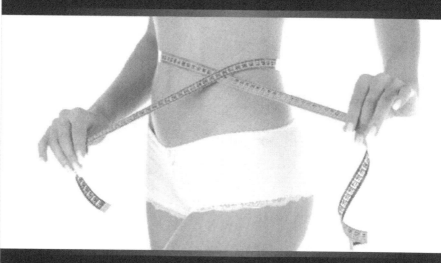

Joseph Correa

Certified Sports Nutritionist

95
Bodybuilder
Meal and Shake
Recipes to Improve
Muscle Growth
Less Work and Faster Results

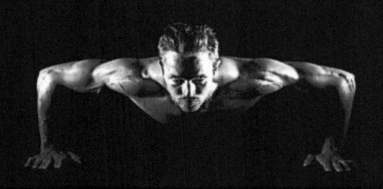

Joseph Correa
Certified Sports Nutritionist

50

Bodybuilder

Shakes to Increase Muscle Mass
High Protein Content in Every Shake

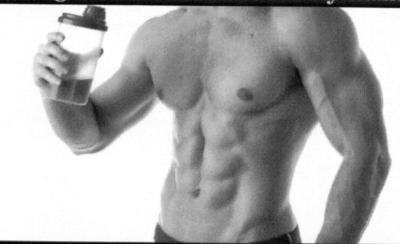

Joseph Correa
Certified Sports Nutritionist

35

Recipes to Lower Your High Blood Pressure

Watch Your Blood Pressure Go Down in Just 7 Days

Joseph Correa
Certified Sports Nutritionist

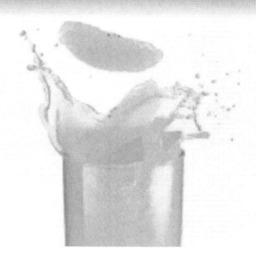

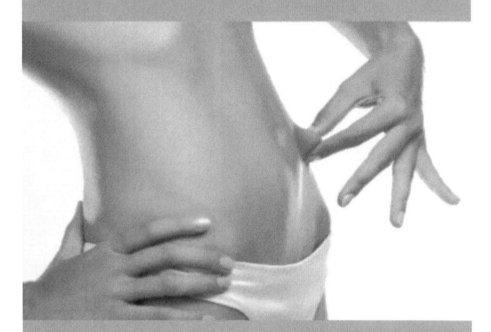

40 WEIGHT LOSS RECIPES FOR A BUSY LIFESTYLE

FOR A BUSY LIFESTYLE

40

THE SOLUTION TO DEALING WITH FAT

Joseph Correa

Certified Sports Nutritionist

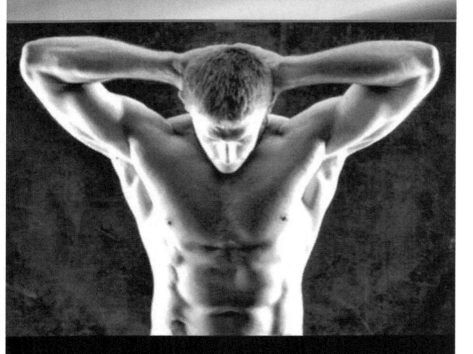

45 BODYBUILDER MEAL RECIPES

INCREASE MUSCLE MASS IN 10 DAYS OR LESS!

Joseph Correa
Certified Sports Nutritionist

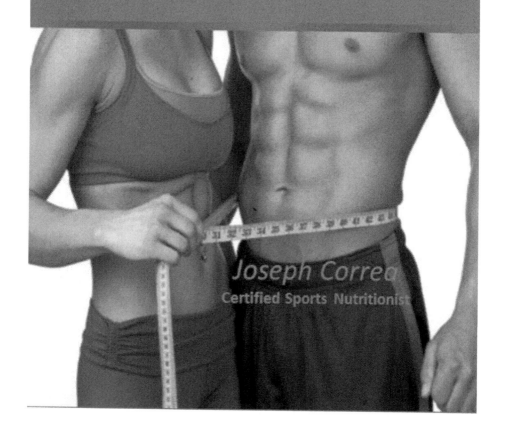

WEIGHT LOSS JUICE RECIPES TO FIGHT OBESITY NOW:

JUICE CLEANSE TO DETOXIFY THE BODY

Joseph Correa

Certified Sports Nutritionist

50

Juice Recipes to Lower Your Blood Pressure

An Easy Way to Reduce High Blood Pressure

Joseph Correa

Certified Sports Nutritionist

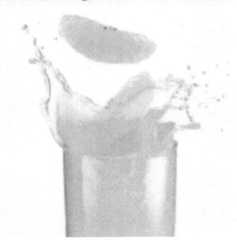

50 Weight Loss Juice Recipes

Juice Recipes

for Body Cleansing
Lose Weight Fast Before Your
Wedding, Party, or Special Event

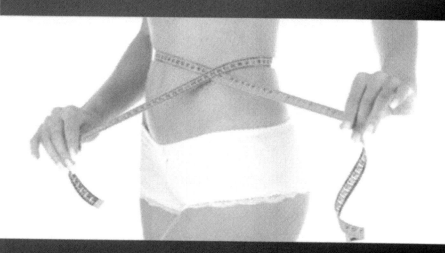

Joseph Correa
Certified Sports Nutritionist

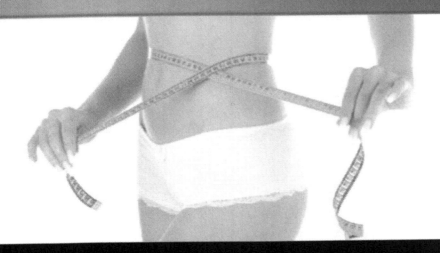

50 Weight Loss Juices

Look Thinner in 10 Days or Less!

Joseph Correa
Certified Sports Nutritionist

55 CANCER PREVENTING
AND CANCER FIGHTING JUICE RECIPES:

BOOST YOUR IMMUNE SYSTEM, IMPROVE YOUR DIGESTION, AND BECOME HEALTHIER TODAY

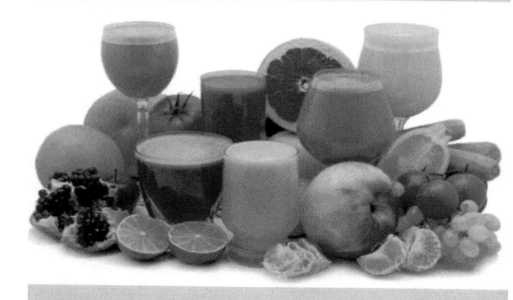

Joseph Correa
Certified Sports Nutritionist

85

Meal and Juice Recipes to Lower Your

High Blood Pressure

Solve Your Hypertension Problem in 12 Days or Less!

Joseph Correa
Certified Sports Nutritionist

90
Weight Loss
Meal and Juice
Recipes to Get Rid of Fat Today!
The Solution to Melting Fat Away Fast!

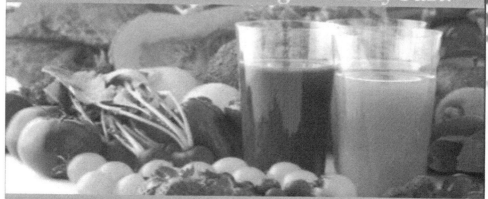

Joseph Correa
Certified Sports Nutritionist

50304873R00083